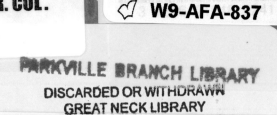

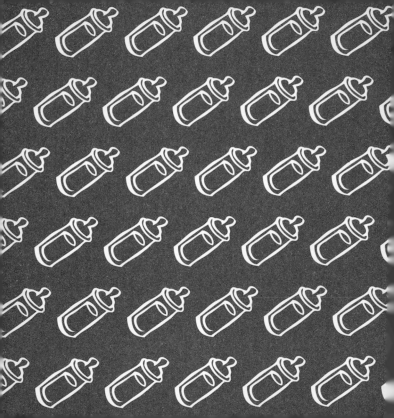

Baby

help.

Tips
for
Grand
parents

Simon Brett

summersdale

Illustrations by
Alex Hallatt

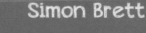

BABY TIPS FOR GRANDPARENTS

This edition published 2012

First published in 2006

Illustrations by Alex Hallatt

Summersdale Publishers Ltd
46 West Street
Chichester
West Sussex
PO19 1RP
UK

www.summersdale.com

Printed and bound in China

ISBN: 978-1-84953-284-6

Substantial discounts on bulk quantities of Summersdale books are available to corporations, professional associations and other organisations. For details contact Summersdale Publishers by telephone: +44 (0) 1243 771107, fax: +44 (0) 1243 786300 or email: nicky@summersdale.com.

To...

From...

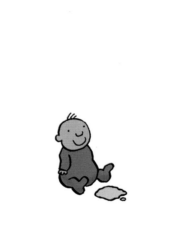

Contents

Introduction

You may think being a grandparent's easy, that all you have to do is sit back and enjoy watching the development of another generation. But being a grandparent brings all kinds of new challenges. It puts new stresses on your relationship with your children and it's also a diplomatic minefield. You'll find, in your new role, you spend a lot of time biting your tongue to avoid saying the wrong thing.

Oh yes, it's tough. How fortunate then that you have this small book of advice to guide you through the choppy waters ahead.

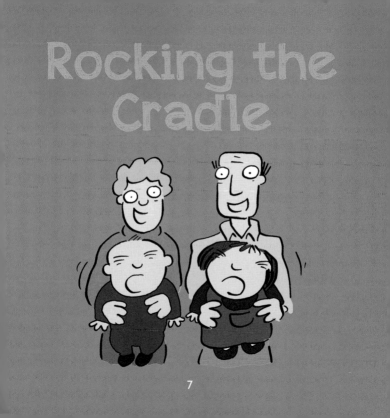

Rocking the Cradle

Before the baby's born:

Try not to ask: 'Should you be doing that in your condition?'

Before the baby's born:

A grandmother-to-be
should try to avoid
turning into a primitive
Wise Woman, dangling keys
or needles over the bump
to predict gender.

9

When its parents announce the name they have chosen for your grandchild, try not to wince – or, even worse, giggle.

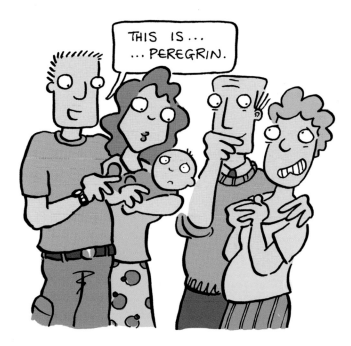

Before the baby's born:

Don't suggest lending your books on pregnancy to the mum-to-be. Fashions in such matters have changed, and the gurus whose advice you followed have been long since discredited.

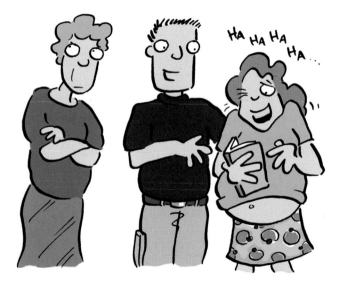

Before the baby's born:

If you want to retain any
friends, try occasionally
to talk to them about
something other than the
impending birth.

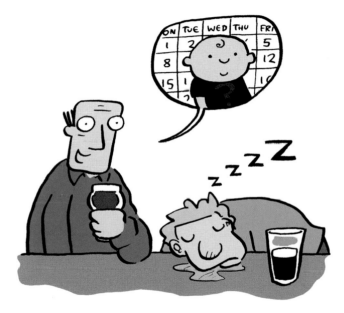

Before the baby's born:

Don't say to first-time parents-to-be, 'You'd better make the most of your freedom now. You won't have any social life once the baby's arrived.' It's true, but there's no point in depressing them before it happens.

What not to say as
a grandparent:

Avoid sentences which
begin, 'I always gave you...'
and end, '... and you've
turned out all right.'

What not to say as a grandparent:

Try to avoid saying, 'In our
day we just got on with it.'

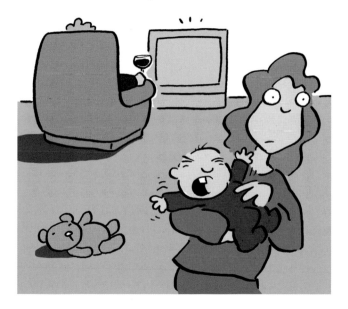

What not to say as a grandparent:

Or, 'The odd non-organic
vegetable never hurt
anyone.'

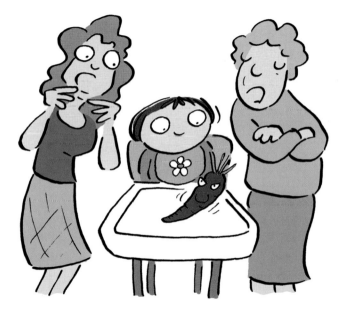

What not to say as a grandparent:

Or, 'We didn't bother with any of that nonsense when you were a baby.'

What not to say as a grandparent:

Never say to a first-time mum-to-be, 'You won't have time to be so fussy with the next one.' While undoubtedly true, it is not what she wants to hear.

What not to say as a grandparent:

When your grandchild
misbehaves, do not
overreact by announcing,
'I'm going to change
my will.'

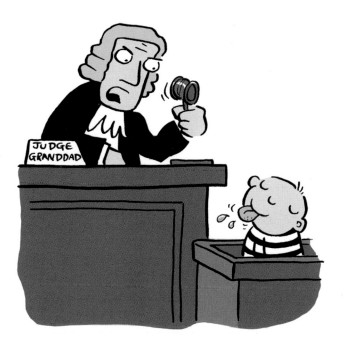

Unavoidable clichés:

'I'm so much more relaxed with them than I was with my own.'

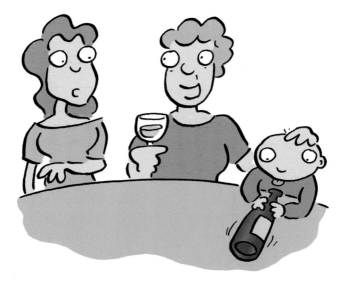

'The trouble is, these days children aren't allowed to have a childhood.'

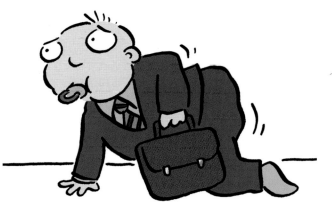

Unavoidable clichés:

'It seems no time at all
since their parents were
that age.'

30

'Ooh, look, the baby's more interested in the wrapping paper than the present!'

Unavoidable clichés:

'Well, you're eating
for two.'

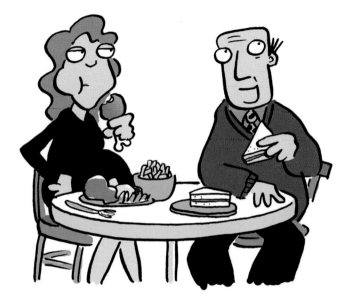

Unavoidable clichés:

'The good thing is you can give them back at the end of the day.'

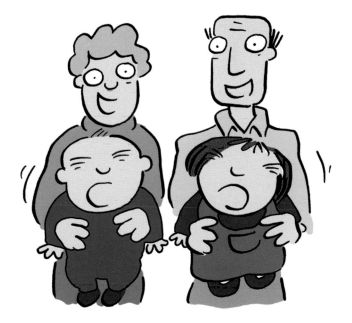

General Rules

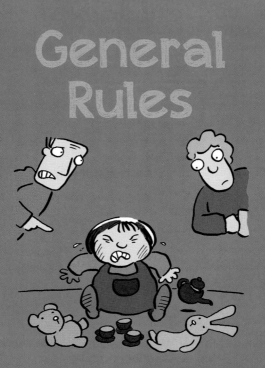

Top tips:

Never pretend you're too
young to be a grandparent.
The contradictory evidence
is there in the cot.

Always deny that there is any rivalry between you and the other set of grandparents. Though, of course, there is.

Top tips:

Do not get down on
the floor to play with your
grandchild unless you are
confident you will be
able to get up again
without assistance.

Even though you've failed with two generations, don't try to realise your dreams through a third.

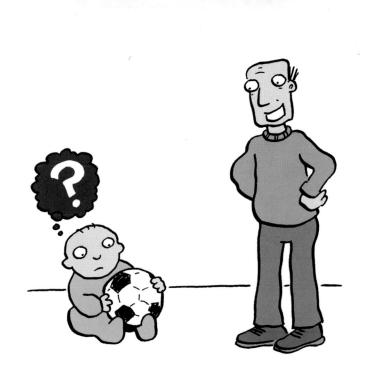

Top tips:

You will meet a lot of
pathetic souls labouring
under the delusion that
their grandchildren
are more beautiful and
intelligent than yours.
Ignore them — obviously
they are wrong.

42

When your grandchildren
come to stay:

When its parents leave
your grandchild at your
house, there are bound to
be tears. But you just have
to pull yourself together.

When your grandchildren
come to stay:

Grandchildren will never
remember where to put
their toys away but they'll
always remember where
you keep the crisps
and biscuits.

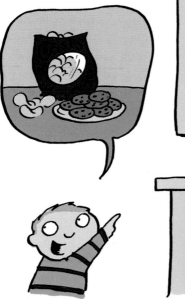
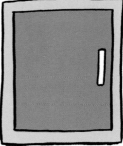
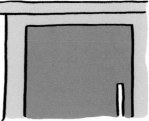

When your grandchildren
come to stay:

If your grandchild can
crawl, remember to move
breakable items out of its
reach (and don't forget
that a baby's reach can
defy the laws of physics).

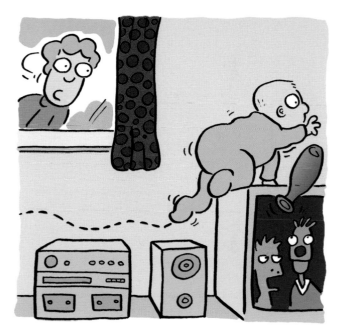

When your grandchildren come to stay:

Having watched you putting DVDs in the machine's tray your grandchildren will be anxious to follow your example. Do not leave any round flat objects lying about – e.g. shortbread circles, Wagon Wheels, mini pizzas...

When your grandchildren
come to stay:

Early nights are very
important when your
grandchild comes to stay.
In order to survive, you
should probably be in bed
by about eight.

49

When your grandchildren
come to stay:

There is an unalterable law
with babies. However fast
asleep they may have been
when they were left in
their grandparents' care,
within five minutes of their
parents' departure they
will be screaming.

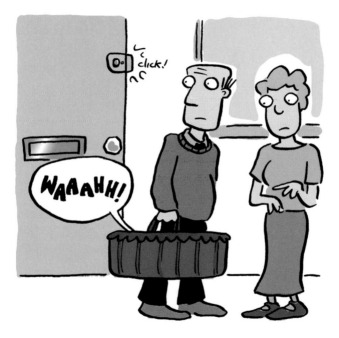

When your grandchildren
come to stay:

If your grandchildren come
to stay with you during
potty training, make sure
you know the expressions
which mean they want to
go. This will save on your
carpet-cleaning bill.

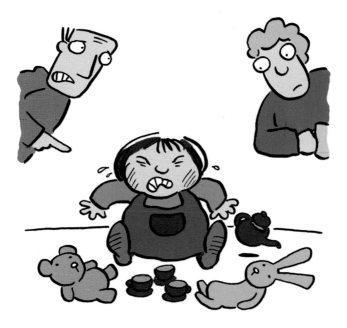

When your grandchildren
come to stay:

Though obviously you
want all your friends and
neighbours to see your
grandchild, remember it is
not a performing animal and
may not do all its tricks
to order.

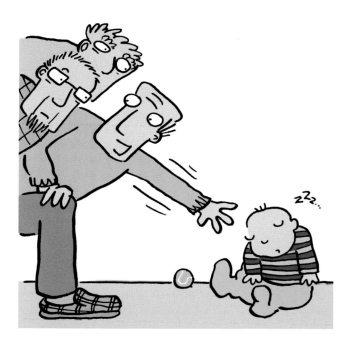

Some disappointing facts:

Not every grandchild who does awfully good finger-painting will turn out to be the next Michelangelo.

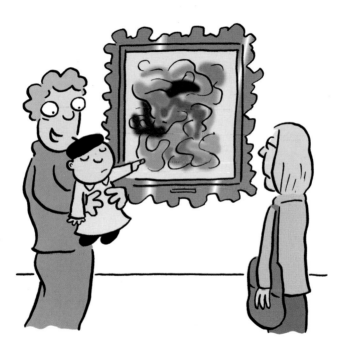

Nor does every baby who looks quite cute go on to become a supermodel.

Nor does every infant who is very good as an ox or ass in the school nativity play go on to become a Hollywood star.

Some disappointing facts:

Remarkable though it
may seem, the progress of
your grandchild's potty
training is not a topic of
universal interest.

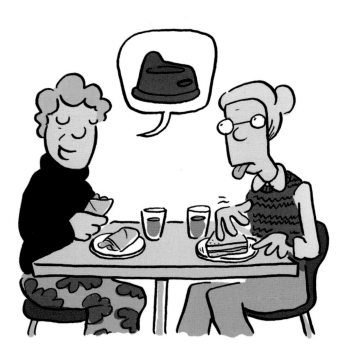

Family Occasions

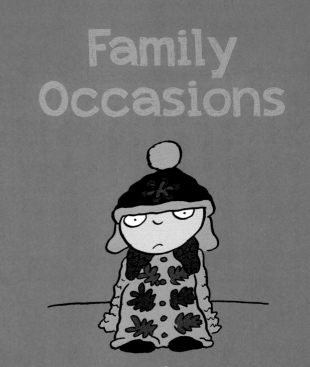

Picture perfect:

Every now and then allow
your grandchild to do
something without taking a
photograph of it.

Picture perfect:

Carry photographs to show at all times. People who claim not to be as interested in your grandchildren as you are must be joking.

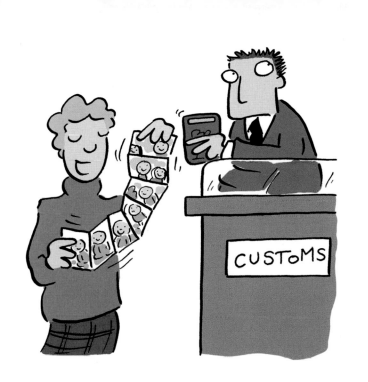

Picture perfect:

You can spend a very long time with your camera poised, waiting for a smile. And when you finally do press the shutter, you almost always miss it.

Picture perfect:

The invention of digital cameras means you don't have to get whole reels developed before you realise that your grandchild isn't smiling in any of the photos.

Picture perfect:

Babies don't understand
the concept of pointing. If
you want them to look in a
certain direction, make
a noise.

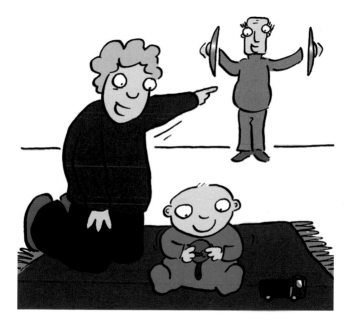

Picture perfect:

Don't embarrass your grandchildren by knitting for them. Unsuitable garments may not last, but photographs do.

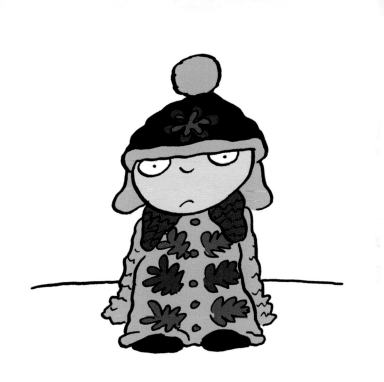

Picture perfect:

It is the obligation of every grandparent with a mobile phone to have a picture of a grandchild as wallpaper. This will mean that you coo every time you turn your phone on.

Presents:

If you do give a grandchild money, do not expect to get away with giving less the next time. They all have little calculators in their brains.

Be very careful when buying clothes for your grandchild's dolls. Giving the wrong garment can destroy your street cred forever.

Presents:

Don't give your grandchild
a present every time you
see it. Every now and then
play hard to get.

75

Presents:

It is astonishing the young
age at which grandchildren
will appreciate a gift
of money.

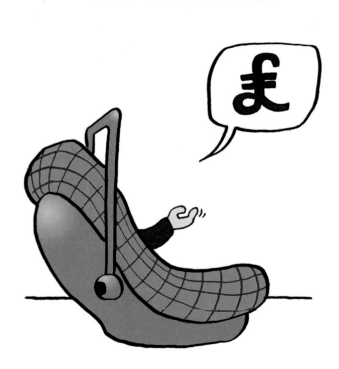

Presents:

If you give your grandchild
a present and get no
thanks, avoid the instinct
to ask, 'What do you say?'
The child is quite likely
to reply, 'Can I have
another one?'

Presents:

From a child's point of view
the word 'educational' on a
toy is the kiss of death.

79

Many parents disapprove of their children being given toy guns. No children do.

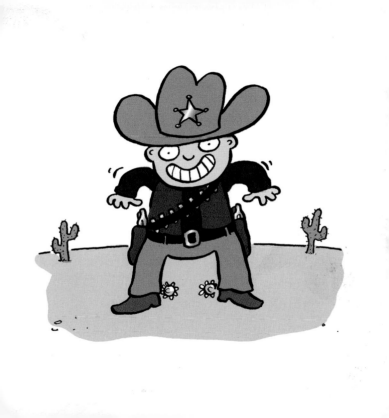

Giving your grandchildren presents that make irritating noises is not fair on their parents... but it is quite fun.

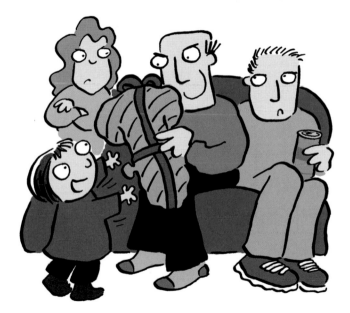

Don't worry if your grandchild ignores your present and plays with the one given by the other set of grandparents: it plays with yours when they visit.

Nursery
Rhymes

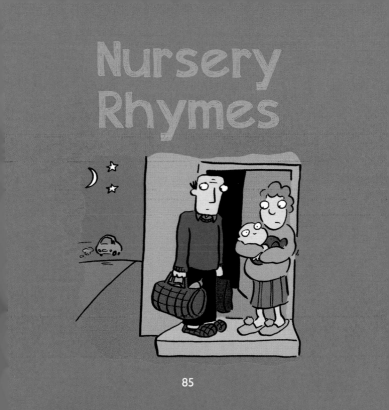

Nursery Rhymes:

You probably grew up with nursery rhymes, but today's children are not so likely to hear them. It is therefore important that you keep the tradition alive. Some of the old rhymes, though, may need a little updating, as in these examples...

Jack Sprat could eat no fat,
His wife could eat no lean;
And so he put her on a diet -
Obesity's obscene.

Nursery Rhymes:

Ding, dong, bell,
Pussy's in the well.
Who put her in?
One of those nasty children
who you must never
play with.

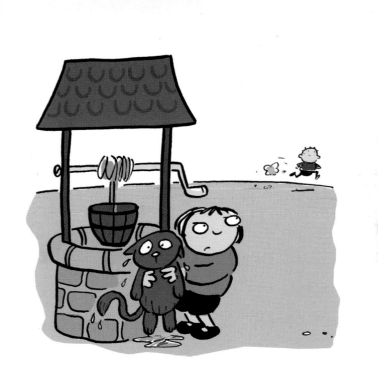

Old King Cole
Was a merry old soul,
And a merry old soul
was he,
He called for his pipe,
To the pub took a stroll,
But he couldn't smoke in
The Fiddlers Three.

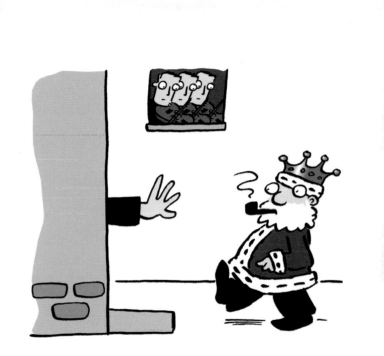

Nursery Rhymes:

Jack and Jill went up
the hill
To fetch a pail of water.
Jack fell down and broke
his crown,
And sued Jill for
negligence after.

Mary, Mary, quite contrary,
How does your
garden grow?
With silver bells, and
cockle shells,
And lots of other stuff
recommended in a
television gardening show.

A final thought...

Never say, 'I'm not just a cheap babysitting service.' The fact is, you are.

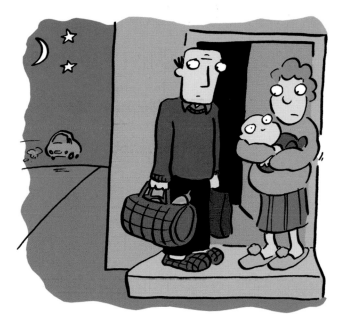

If you're interested in finding out more
about our humour books follow us
on Twitter: **@SummersdaleLOL**

www.summersdale.com